The Handbook for Supporting Mental and Emotional Well-Being

The Importance of Supporting Your Mental and Emotional Well-Being

Mental and emotional well-being is essential to overall health and happiness. It refers to a state of being in which an individual is able to cope with the normal stresses of life, work productively, and make a positive contribution to their community. When we have good mental and emotional well-being, we are better able to make healthy choices, form positive relationships, and handle difficult situations.

Mental and emotional well-being also plays a critical role in physical health. Chronic stress, for example, has been linked to a variety of physical health problems, including heart disease, diabetes, and obesity. Additionally, mental health conditions such as anxiety and depression can lead to a variety of physical symptoms. By addressing our mental and emotional well-being, we can improve our physical health as well.

Good mental and emotional well-being can also improve our relationships and interactions with others. When we are feeling mentally and emotionally well, we are more likely to be patient, understanding, and empathetic. This can lead to better relationships with friends and family, as well as improved interactions in the workplace.

Mental and emotional well-being is also closely linked to our ability to learn, grow and achieve our goals. When we are feeling mentally and emotionally well, we are more likely to be motivated and engaged in our work, studies and hobbies. This can lead to improved performance, satisfaction, and a sense of accomplishment.

Finally, mental and emotional well-being is essential for overall health and happiness, it plays a critical role in physical health, improves our relationships and interactions with others, and helps us to achieve our goals and reach our full potential. It is important to take care of our mental and emotional well-being and seek help if we need it, as this can lead to a happier, healthier and more fulfilling life.

Self-Care

Self-care refers to the actions and practices individuals engage in to take care of their physical, mental, and emotional well-being. It is a proactive approach to maintaining and improving one's overall health and well-being. Self-care involves identifying one's needs and taking steps to meet those needs in a consistent and ongoing way.

There are many different forms of self-care, and what works for one person may not work for another. Some examples of self-care activities include:

- Eating a healthy diet
- Exercise and physical activity
- Getting enough sleep

- Practicing mindfulness and meditation
- Reading or engaging in a hobby
- Spending time outdoors
- Keeping a journal or writing down one's thoughts
- Setting boundaries and saying "no" to demands that are not in line with one's values and goals

Self-care is an important aspect of overall well-being and it is especially important during times of stress or change. It helps to improve our mood, reduce anxiety and depression, lower the risk of chronic diseases, and improve our overall physical and mental health. It also allows us to better cope with the demands of daily life, and it helps us to be more resilient in the face of stressors and challenges.

It is important to note that self-care is not selfish, it is a necessary aspect of maintaining our well-being, it is not a luxury but a necessity. It is not something that we do occasionally but it's a regular and consistent practice that should be integrated into our daily routine.

In summary, self-care is a proactive and ongoing approach to taking care of one's physical, mental and emotional well-being, it involves identifying one's needs and taking steps to meet those needs in a consistent and ongoing way. It helps to improve our mood, reduce anxiety and depression, lower the risk of chronic diseases, and improve our overall physical and mental health, while building our resilience in the face of adversity.

Self-Care Activities

It can't be stressed enough that what works for one person may not work for another. But it's important to have a place to start. Consider these 25 different self-care activities and how you might incorporate a few of them into your daily routine:

1. **Eating** a healthy diet that includes a variety of fruits, vegetables, whole grains, and lean proteins.
2. **Engaging** in regular physical activity such as jogging, cycling, swimming, yoga, or weightlifting.
3. **Getting** enough sleep each night, aiming for 7-9 hours of sleep per night.

4. **Practicing** mindfulness through meditation, deep breathing exercises, or yoga.

5. **Reading** for pleasure or engaging in a hobby such as painting, writing, or playing a musical instrument.

6. **Spending** time outdoors, whether it be going for a walk, hike, or simply sitting in nature.

7. **Keeping** a journal or writing down one's thoughts and feelings.

8. **Setting** boundaries and saying "no" to demands that are not in line with one's values and goals.

9. **Practicing** self-compassion and being kind to oneself.

10. **Engaging** in regular self-reflection and introspection.

11. **Listening** to music or podcast.

12. **Learning** something new or taking a class.

13. **Volunteering** or giving back to the community.

14. **Practicing** gratitude and positive thinking.

15. **Getting** a massage or visiting a spa.

16. **Planning** a vacation or a trip.

17. **Getting** a pet.

18. **Spending** quality time with loved ones.

19. **Practicing** good hygiene and grooming.

20. **Doing** something creative like cooking or baking.

21. **Having** a relaxing bath or shower.

22. **Taking** a nap or a power nap.

23. **Organizing** or decluttering your space.

24. **Watching** a comedy or a favorite movie.

25. **Get** a good book and cuddle up with a blanket.

It's important to note that self-care activities will vary from person to person and what works for one person may not work for another. It's important to find what works best for you, and make self-care a regular and consistent practice in your life. Also, it's important to seek professional help if you find difficulty in maintaining your mental and emotional well-being, as well as physical health.

The Impact of Stress

Stress is the body's response to any demand or threat, perceived or real. It is a natural and normal reaction to certain events or circumstances in our lives. Stress can be caused by a wide range of things, such as work-related problems, financial difficulties, relationship issues, health concerns, or major life changes.

When we experience stress, our bodies release hormones such as adrenaline and cortisol, which prepare us to respond to the perceived threat or demand. This is commonly known as the "fight or flight" response. This response is helpful in situations where we need to take quick action, such as in an emergency. However, when we are constantly exposed to stressors, the continuous release of these hormones can have negative effects on our physical and mental health.

Acute stress is a short-term stress that occurs in response to a specific event or situation, such as a job interview or a car accident. Acute stress typically subsides once the event is over, or the situation is resolved.

Chronic stress, on the other hand, is long-term stress that occurs in response to ongoing or unresolved stressors, such as a demanding job, financial difficulties, or a difficult relationship. Chronic stress can have a significant impact on our physical and mental health, and can increase the risk of developing various health conditions such as heart disease, diabetes, and depression. Chronic stress can also exacerbate existing mental health conditions, making them more difficult to manage.

Symptoms of stress can vary from person to person and can include physical symptoms such as headaches, fatigue, muscle tension, and changes in appetite, as well as emotional symptoms such as anxiety, irritability, and depression.

Stress can also lead to changes in our behavior such as overeating, smoking, alcohol and drug abuse, which can further impact our mental and emotional well-being. It can also impact our ability to think clearly, make decisions, and remember things. This can make it difficult to perform well at work or school, and can make it harder to form and maintain relationships. It can affect our sleep patterns, leading to insomnia or difficulty falling asleep which can exacerbate the mental and emotional symptoms. Stress can also weaken the immune system, making it harder for our bodies to fight off infections and illnesses, which can further impact our overall health and well-being.

It's important to note that while stress is a normal and natural response, it's important to manage stress effectively in order to maintain our well-being. This can include identifying and addressing the sources of stress, practicing self-care, and seeking professional help if needed.

In summary, stress is the body's response to any demand or threat, perceived or real. It can be caused by a wide range of things, and can have negative effects on our physical and mental health when it becomes chronic. It's important to manage stress effectively in order to maintain our well-being by identifying and addressing the sources of stress, practicing self-care, and seeking professional help if needed.

Managing Stress

Many of the self-care activities mentioned earlier are applicable when managing stress and reworded below to expand on some of those suggestions. Below you will find a few more activities that could also help to manage stress, but ultimately, it is up to each individual to find what works for themselves and to incorporate those practices daily to help manage stress:

Deep breathing exercises: This technique helps to slow down the heart rate and lower blood pressure, which can help to reduce feelings of stress and anxiety.

Time management: Prioritizing tasks and managing time effectively can help to reduce feelings of overwhelm and stress.

Mindfulness: Mindfulness techniques such as meditation and yoga can help to improve focus and reduce feelings of stress and anxiety.

Exercise: Regular physical activity can help to reduce stress and improve overall mental and physical health.

Relaxation techniques: Techniques such as progressive muscle relaxation, guided imagery, and self-hypnosis can help to reduce feelings of stress and tension.

Social support: Talking to friends and family, or seeking support from a therapist or counselor can help to reduce feelings of stress and isolation.

Journaling: Writing down one's thoughts and feelings can help to process and release emotions, and can be a useful tool for managing stress.

Humor: Laughing and finding humor in situations can help to reduce stress and improve overall mood.

Prioritizing self-care: Engaging in regular self-care activities such as exercise, eating a healthy diet, and getting enough sleep can help to improve overall well-being and reduce stress.

Identifying and addressing the source of stress: Identifying the source of stress and taking steps to address it can help to reduce and manage stress effectively.

Mindful eating: Eating mindfully and paying attention to the food we eat, can help to reduce stress and improve overall well-being.

Listen to music or podcasts: Listening to music or a podcast can distract, relax and enhance your mood from those sources of stressors in your life.

Take a break: Taking regular breaks throughout the day can help to reduce feelings of stress and improve overall productivity.

Take a walk in nature: Being in nature can help to reduce feelings of stress and anxiety by providing a sense of calm and tranquility. Being around natural elements such as plants and trees can have a grounding effect and can remind us of our connection to the natural world.

Practice gratitude and positive thinking: Incorporating a purposeful daily mindset can help reduce and manage your stress

Get a massage or visit a spa: Make physical self-care a consistent practice to help reduce and manage your stress

Engage in a hobby or learn something new: It can be anything. Think back to when you were a kid, and those passions or thoughts you used to daydream about. Discover them for the first time, rediscover them again, but find something that keeps your mind focused on learning something new or developing something you love to do.

Get a pet: Having a pet can be a great source of stress relief. Pets can help release the 'feel good' hormone oxytocin through physical touch. They provide companionship, a sense of responsibility, improved mood through the release of endorphins which act as natural pain killers for the body, as well as a great source of pure joy and laughter.

Seek professional help: Talking to a therapist or counselor can help to address the underlying causes of stress and develop coping strategies.

It's important to note that different techniques may work better for different people, it's important to experiment with different techniques and find what works best for you. It's also important to seek professional help if you find difficulty in managing stress.

Deep Breathing Exercises for Managing Stress

Deep breathing exercises are a simple and effective way to manage stress. Here are a few examples of deep breathing exercises that you can try:

Diaphragmatic breathing: Sit or lie down in a comfortable position and place one hand on your chest and the other on your belly. Inhale deeply through your nose, allowing your belly to rise as you fill your lungs with air. Exhale slowly through your mouth, allowing your belly to fall.

4-7-8 breathing: Exhale completely through your mouth, then inhale quietly through your nose to a mental count of four. Hold your breath for a count of seven. Exhale completely through your mouth to a count of eight.

Box breathing: Sit or lie down in a comfortable position. Inhale for a count of four, hold your breath for a count of four, exhale for a count of four, and hold your breath again for a count of four before repeating.

Alternate Nostril Breathing: Sit comfortably and using your right thumb, close your right nostril. Inhale through your left nostril, then use your ring finger to close your left nostril and release your thumb to exhale through your right nostril. Repeat the process, inhaling through your right nostril and exhaling through your left nostril.

Belly breathing: Sit or lie down in a comfortable position. Place one hand on your chest and the other on your belly.

Inhale deeply, allowing your belly to rise as you fill your lungs with air. Exhale slowly, allowing your belly to fall.

It's important to practice deep breathing exercises regularly in order to see the benefits. You can practice deep breathing exercises for a few minutes a day, or as needed when you feel stressed. It's also important to find a comfortable place and position to practice the deep breathing exercise.

Relaxation Techniques for Managing Stress

Relaxation techniques are a great way to manage and reduce stress. Here are a few examples of relaxation techniques that you can try out on your own:

Progressive muscle relaxation (PMR): This technique involves tensing and then relaxing different muscle groups in the body, starting at the feet and working up to the head. This can help to release tension and reduce feelings of stress and anxiety.

Guided imagery: This technique involves using your imagination to visualize a peaceful scene or place, such as a beach or a forest. This can help to reduce feelings of stress and anxiety by providing a mental escape from the stressors of daily life.

Self-hypnosis: This technique involves using hypnosis to relax the mind and body and reduce feelings of stress and anxiety.

Yoga: Yoga is a form of physical and mental exercise that can help to reduce stress and improve overall well-being.

Tai Chi: Tai Chi is a martial art that involves slow, flowing movements and deep breathing. It is a gentle form of exercise that can help to reduce stress and improve overall well-being.

Meditation: Meditation is a practice that involves sitting quietly and focusing on the present moment. It can help to reduce feelings of stress and anxiety by promoting mindfulness and relaxation.

Autogenic training: This technique involves repeating specific phrases and focusing on sensations in your body, such as warmth or heaviness, in order to relax and reduce stress. A possible phrase to use is, "Every day, and in every way, I am getting better and better". Say that a dozen times before going to bed and when waking up and watch your mood enhance over the course of a few weeks of practice.

Acupuncture: Acupuncture is a traditional Chinese medicine technique that involves the insertion of thin needles into specific points on the body. This can help to reduce stress and improve overall well-being. Please find a trained professional to discover the benefits of acupuncture.

It's important to experiment with different relaxation techniques and find what works best for you. It's also important to practice relaxation techniques regularly in order to see the benefits.

Mindfully Eating

Eating mindfully involves paying attention to the act of eating and being present in the moment while eating. Here are a few ways to practice mindful eating:

Set aside time for eating: Designate specific times for meals and snacks, and avoid eating while doing other activities such as watching TV or working.

Slow down: Take your time while eating, chew your food slowly, and savor the flavors and textures of the food.

Pay attention to hunger and fullness cues: Pay attention to your body's signals of hunger and fullness, and eat when you are hungry and stop when you are full.

Eliminate distractions: Avoid eating in front of screens or while doing other activities.

Engage all your senses: Take time to notice the colors, smells, and textures of your food.

Show gratitude: Before you start eating, take a moment to show gratitude for the food you have and the people who have helped to produce it.

Practice mindful eating regularly: Make mindful eating a regular habit, try to do it at least once a day, and gradually increase the frequency.

Be kind to yourself: It's okay to slip up, don't be hard on yourself if you find it difficult to eat mindfully, keep practicing.

Remember that mindful eating is a skill that can be learned and practiced over time, it's not something that you will be able to do perfectly right away. It's important to be patient with yourself and to keep practicing.

Practicing Gratitude and Positive Thinking

Practicing gratitude and positive thinking can be a powerful tool for managing and reducing stress. Here are a few ways to practice gratitude and positive thinking:

Keep a gratitude journal: Write down a few things that you are grateful for each day. This can help to shift your focus from negative thoughts to positive ones.

Practice mindfulness: Take a few minutes each day to focus on the present moment and appreciate what you have, rather than dwelling on what you lack.

Practice positive affirmations: Repeat positive phrases to yourself such as "I am strong," "I am capable," or "I am worthy." This can help to shift negative thoughts to positive ones.

Find the good in difficult situations:
Try to find the silver lining in difficult
situations, rather than focusing on the
negative aspects.

Show gratitude to others: Show
appreciation to the people in your life,
whether it's through words, actions, or
small gestures.

Do something kind for someone else:
Helping others can be a great way to shift
focus from one's own problems to the well-
being of others, and it can also be a way to
show gratitude.

Be thankful for the small things:
Practice being grateful for the small
things in life, such as a warm bed, a good
meal, or a sunny day.

Practice visualization: Imagine yourself
in a positive situation, visualize it in your

mind as vividly as possible, feeling the emotions and sensations as if it were real.

It's important to remember that practicing gratitude and positive thinking is a skill that takes time and practice to develop, it's not something that will happen overnight. It's also important to remember that it's normal to have negative thoughts and feelings, it's not about eliminating them but to shift the balance towards the positive thoughts.

The Importance of Having a Support System

Having a support system is important for maintaining mental and emotional well-being, as well as for coping with stress and other challenges. A support system can consist of friends, family, or professional help. Here are a few reasons why having a support system is important:

Emotional support: Having people to talk to about your feelings, thoughts and worries can provide emotional support, which can help to reduce feelings of stress, anxiety, and isolation.

Social support: Having people to spend time with can provide social support, which can help to improve overall well-being, reduce stress, and improve mental health.

Problem-solving assistance: Having a support system can help you to find solutions to problems, to get different perspectives on a situation, and to take action on finding solutions.

Encouragement and motivation: A support system can provide encouragement and motivation to pursue goals, and to make positive changes in one's life.

Sense of belonging: Having a support system can provide a sense of belonging and connectedness, which can help to improve overall well-being and reduce feelings of stress and isolation.

Professional help: A support system can also include professional help, such as a therapist, counselor, or coach, who can provide guidance and support in addressing mental health issues and coping with stress.

It's important to note that the support system can take different forms and different people may have different preferences. It's important to find the right support system that works for you. It's also important to remember that it's okay to reach out for help, it's a sign of strength rather than weakness.

Building a Support System

Building a support system can take time, but it's an important step in maintaining mental and emotional well-being. Here are a few ways to build a support system:

Reach out to friends and family: Spend time with people you trust and feel comfortable talking to. Let them know that you value their support and that you are there for them as well.

Join a support group: Join a support group related to your specific needs, whether that's a group for people with a particular health condition, a group for people who are going through a difficult time, or a group for people who share a common interest.

Connect with people online: Join online communities or social media groups related to your specific needs.

Volunteer: Get involved in volunteer activities and organizations. This can be a great way to meet new people and make connections while giving back to your community.

Develop new hobbies and interests: Take up a new hobby or activity, or join a club or class. This can be a great way to meet new people who share your interests.

Seek professional help: Consider seeking professional help such as a therapist, counselor or coach to provide guidance and support in addressing mental health issues and coping with stress.

Make a plan: Make a plan to build your support system and set goals for yourself.

It's important to be proactive in building your support system, and to not be afraid to ask for help.

Keep an open mind: Building a support system can take time, don't be discouraged if it doesn't happen right away, keep an open mind and be persistent, you'll find the right people at the right time.

It's important to have a diverse support system, one that includes different types of people, such as family, friends, professional help, and online communities. This way, you can have different sources of support for different needs. Remember that building a support system is an ongoing process, it's important to keep working on it and to not be afraid to reach out for help.

Professional Support

Professional support, such as therapy or counseling, can be an important component of a support system for managing and reducing stress. Here are a few reasons why professional support is important:

Expertise: Therapists and counselors are trained professionals who have expertise in understanding and addressing mental health issues, stress, and emotional well-being. They can provide guidance and support in addressing specific issues.

Confidentiality: Professional support provides a safe and confidential environment to talk about personal and sensitive issues.

Objectivity: A therapist or counselor can provide an objective perspective on a situation and can help to identify patterns or behaviors that may be contributing to stress or mental health issues.

Evidence-based treatment: Therapy and counseling are evidence-based treatments that have been shown to be effective in addressing mental health issues and reducing stress.

Identifying underlying issues: A therapist or counselor can help to identify underlying issues that may be contributing to stress or mental health issues, and can help to develop strategies for addressing them.

Creating a sense of control: Professional support can help individuals to feel more in control of their thoughts, feelings, and behaviors, which can be an effective way to reduce stress.

Personal growth: Professional support can help individuals to learn new coping skills, gain insight into themselves and their behaviors, and work towards personal growth and self-improvement.

Supportive environment: Professional support provides a supportive and non-judgmental environment where individuals can freely express themselves and receive guidance and support.

It's important to note that therapy and counseling are not one-size-fits-all, different approaches and different therapists may work better for different people, it's important to find the right fit for you. It's also important to remember that professional support is not a sign of weakness, it's a sign of strength to take control of one's mental and emotional well-being.

About the Author

Antonio is a father of two children who he loves dearly. He has been working in the field of education for almost twenty-five years, primarily with students ages K-21. He believes that basic education is the key to supporting more people all over the world. Knowing how to manage your own mental and emotional well-being could alleviate so much suffering in the world. It is his hope that one day every general physician will hand out this handbook to every patient, just so they have the basics to support their own mental and emotional well-being. Education is truly the most powerful tool we have to transform the future.

Disclaimer

Please note that the advice provided is intended for informational purposes only and should not be taken as legal or professional advice. It is important to always seek the guidance of a qualified professional when making decisions that may have legal consequences. Additionally, it is important to use your own judgment and intuition when making any decisions, as ultimately you are responsible for the outcome. Please consult with a qualified professional before making any decisions that may have legal or other significant consequences. This disclaimer is not intended to limit or exclude any liability that may not be excluded or limited by law.

This handbook was a collaboration between the author and an open AI platform, with the sole purpose of helping people all over the world, and by helping to educate everyone to be knowledgeable on how to support their own mental and emotional well-being.

First Edition: 2023
ISBN: 9798373687546

Content Feedback: Please direct all feedback to **www.handbooksforhumanity.com**

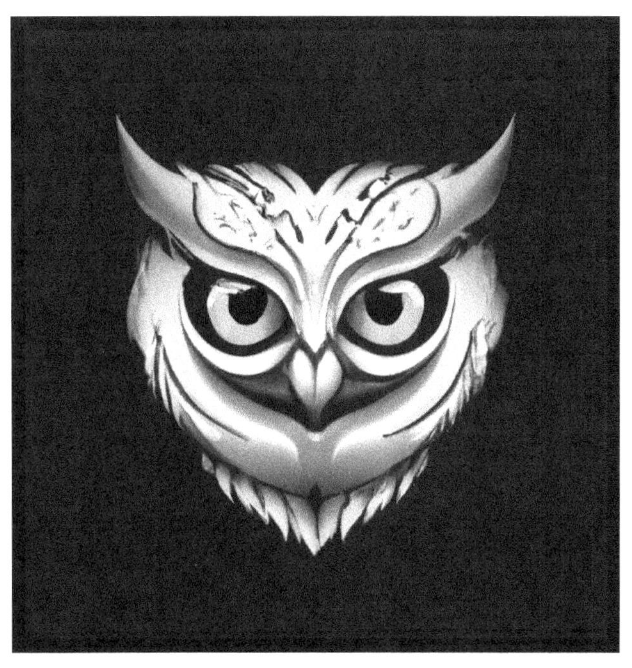

Copyright © 2023
Gufo Publishing